Heart Disease

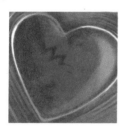

what you should know

**Blackwell
Science**

PKY

Heart Disease

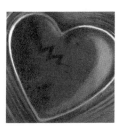

what you should know

Written by Dean J. Kereiakes, MD, FACC,
and Douglas Wetherill, MS
Illustrated by Laura L. Seeley

©2001 by Robertson & Fisher Publishing Company. Second Edition.

Written by: Dean J. Kereiakes, MD, FACC; and Douglas Wetherill, MS
Contributing Editors: Paul Ribisl, PhD; Rona Wharton, MEd, RD, LD; and John Young, MD
Illustrated by: Laura L. Seeley

Distributors:
Blackwell Publishing
c/o AIDC
P.O. Box 20, 50 Winter Sport Lane, Williston, VT 05495-0020 USA
(Telephone orders: 800-216-2522; fax orders: 802-864-7626)

Blackwell Science, Ltd.
c/o Marston Book Services, Ltd.
P.O. Box 269, Abingdon, Oxon OX14 4YN, England
(Telephone orders: 44-01235-465500; fax orders: 44-01235-465555)

Printed in Canada
01 02 03 04 5 4 3 2 1 (ISBN:0-632-04529-9)

The Blackwell Science logo is a trademark of Blackwell Science Ltd., registered at the United Kingdom Trade Marks Registry.

A catalog record for this book is available from the U.S. Library of Congress.

To mom and dad: Morfydd and George

To my sisters: Rona, Sian, and Megan

In memory of my brother: Gareth

"No matter what accomplishments you achieve, somebody helps you."
—*Althea Gibson*

The authors would like to acknowledge the generous support of the following individuals for their input regarding changes to the second edition: John Young, MD; Angela Ginty; and Paul Neff.

Treatment Disclaimer

This book is for education purposes, not for use in the treatment of medical conditions. It is based on skilled medical opinion as of the date of publication. However, medical science advances and changes rapidly. Furthermore, diagnosis and treatment are often complex and involve more than one disease process or medical issue to determine proper care. If you believe you may have a medical condition described in the book, consult your doctor.

Table of Contents

Introduction

Heart disease, especially coronary heart disease, is an everyday part of our culture. It is also the most common cause of death. What can be done to reverse this trend? A large percentage of cardiovascular disease is genetic or inherited. However, there are things you can do to reduce your chance of having a heart attack. You can start by understanding what cardiovascular disease is and making the necessary changes in your life. If you have had a cardiac event, or if you think you may be at risk of cardiovascular disease, **now** is the time to take command of your life.

— Dean and Douglas

Heart Anatomy

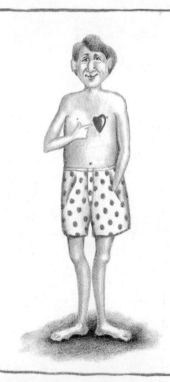

The heart

The heart is a muscle.
It pumps blood to the
head and the body.
It is about the size of
your fist and sits just
to the left of the
middle of your chest.

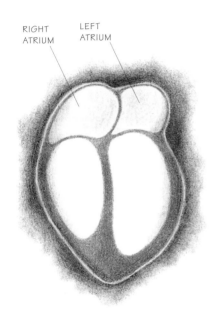

RIGHT ATRIUM

LEFT ATRIUM

The heart is asymmetrical. It is made up of 4 chambers. The top 2 chambers are called the **atria**. The atria collect blood returning to the heart. The atria then dump the blood into the ventricles.

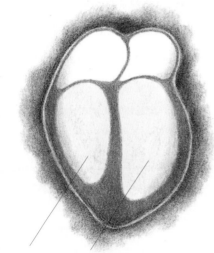

RIGHT
VENTRICLE

LEFT
VENTRICLE

The bottom 2 chambers are called the **ventricles**. The ventricles are larger than the atria, and the left one is more muscular. When the ventricles contract, they force blood out of the heart to different parts of the body.

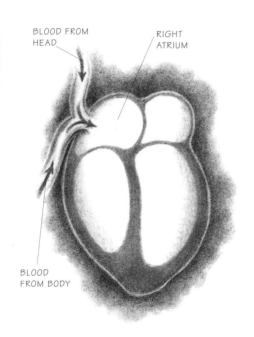

BLOOD FROM HEAD

RIGHT ATRIUM

BLOOD FROM BODY

The body uses nutrients and oxygen carried by the blood. The blood returning to the heart has had oxygen removed. This "deoxygenated" blood collects in the **right atrium**.

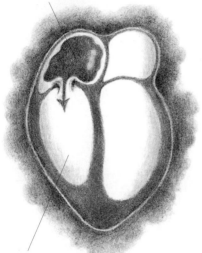

BLOOD FLOWS INTO
RIGHT ATRIUM

RIGHT VENTRICLE
RECEIVES BLOOD
FROM RIGHT ATRIUM

The blood in the
right atrium
goes into the
right ventricle.

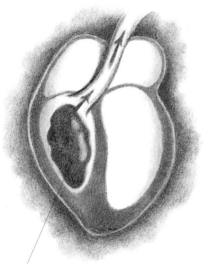

LUNGS

RIGHT VENTRICLE

The **right ventricle** pumps blood to the **lungs** where the blood picks up oxygen.

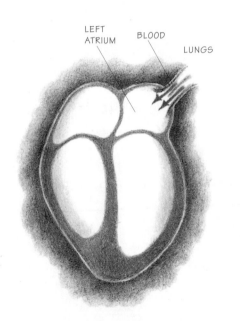

LEFT
ATRIUM   BLOOD

LUNGS

Once the blood picks
up oxygen in the
lungs, it is ready
to be used by
the body again.
The oxygen-rich
blood returns to
the heart and
collects inside the
left atrium.

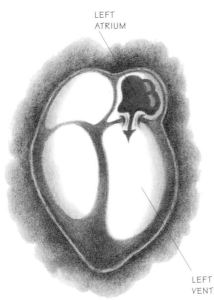

LEFT
ATRIUM

LEFT
VENTRICLE

The **left atrium** contracts and sends the blood to the **left ventricle**.

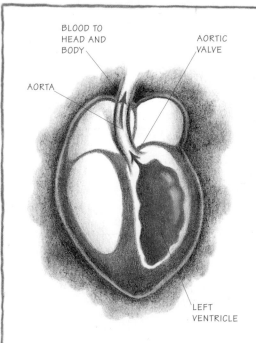

BLOOD TO HEAD AND BODY

AORTIC VALVE

AORTA

LEFT VENTRICLE

The **left ventricle** contracts and pumps oxygenated blood through the **aortic valve** into the **aorta**. The blood then travels through the **aorta,** providing life-sustaining oxygen and nutrients to the body.

So:

1) Blood with lower oxygen content collects in the right atrium.

2) The right ventricle pumps blood to the lungs where it picks up oxygen.

3) Oxygen-rich blood collects in the left atrium.

4) The left ventricle pumps oxygen-rich blood to the head and the rest of the body.

Arteries and Coronary Arteries

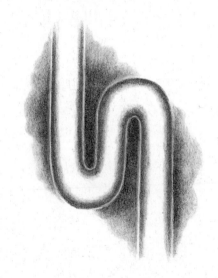

Arteries carry blood
much the same way
a plumbing system
carries water
throughout a house.

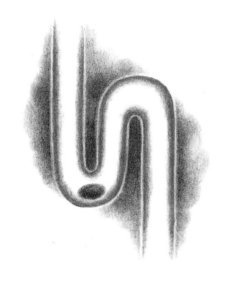

Over time, debris traveling through the pipes may collect in a bend. Debris that collects and restricts water flow is known as a clog or a blockage.

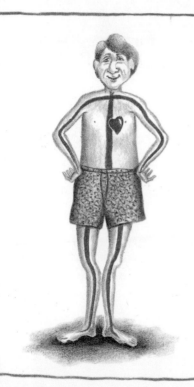

Arteries and veins wind throughout the body carrying blood. Arteries carry blood away from the heart. Veins carry blood back to the heart.

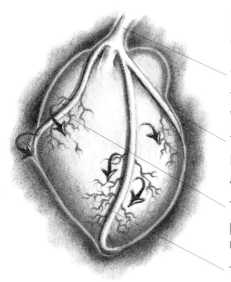

The heart has its own arteries to provide blood to the heart muscle.

The **aorta** supplies blood to the arteries of the heart as well as to the rest of the body.

The **circumflex artery** supplies blood to the lateral or side aspect of the heart.

The **right coronary artery** provides blood to the back or underside of the heart.

The **left anterior descending artery** supplies blood to the front of the heart.

To give you some idea of their size, the **coronary arteries** are only about the size of a strand of spaghetti.

(APPROXIMATE SIZE OF SPAGHETTI)

At birth, the inside of the arteries, including the coronary arteries, is slippery — similar to a nonstick pan. The blood cells (represented by the small cars) flow smoothly through the arteries.

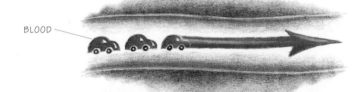

BLOOD

What happens to an artery
during a person's lifetime?

Fatty streaks in the arteries start to develop in the first decade of life as a result of lipids moving into the cell wall of the artery.

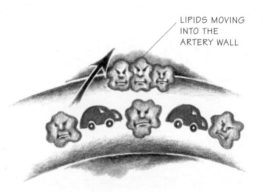

LIPIDS MOVING INTO THE ARTERY WALL

These fatty streaks may become more advanced **atherosclerotic lesions** in the presence of risk factors such as smoking, high blood pressure, obesity, high cholesterol, and physical inactivity. The fatty streaks may then progress to **atheromas** and **fibroatheromas**, which are more "advanced lesions" and are often referred to as **plaque**.

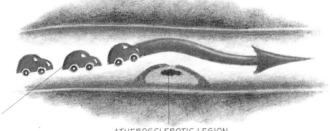

BLOOD

ATHEROSCLEROTIC LESION

Buildups may occur at different points along the length of the artery. Plaque buildups are not limited to the arteries of the heart. They can occur and restrict blood flow in arteries throughout your body.

PLAQUE BUILDUP

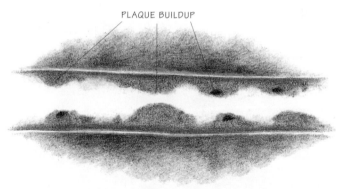

The total blockage of the artery may occur due to: a) the **buildup** of plaque, b) the formation of a blood clot on the plaque, or c) the plaque **rupturing** and causing a larger blood clot to form. The complete blockage of the artery is called an **occlusion**.

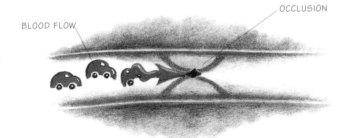

BLOOD FLOW

OCCLUSION

What happens if an artery becomes completely blocked?

An artery that is completely blocked has no blood flowing through it. If the heart muscle does not receive blood, then it does not receive nutrients and oxygen.

When the heart does not receive oxygen, it experiences **ischemia**. This may result in **heart pain** (angina) or a **heart attack**. Ischemia, if prolonged and severe enough, may cause a portion of the heart muscle to die (heart attack).

LACK OF BLOOD FLOW

BLOCKAGE

What are some symptoms of a possible heart attack?

- **Angina**, or heart pain, usually felt as a pressure, ache, tightness, squeezing, or **burning sensation** under the breastbone and often extending to the neck, jaw, shoulders, or down the arm (most frequently the left arm)
- **Nausea**
- **Shortness of breath** and/or **sweating**

Interestingly, **diabetic patients** do not "feel" angina in the same way and are more than twice as likely as nondiabetics to have a "silent" or unrecognized heart attack.

25

Quite often, people who are having a heart attack say they feel like "an elephant is standing on my chest."

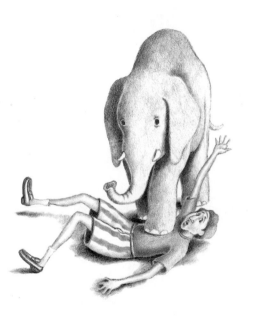

Preventing coronary artery disease

What can be done to reduce your chances of developing heart disease? Generally, cardiovascular disease takes a long time to develop. You may reduce your chances of developing heart disease by changing certain habits or "risk factors."

Risk Factors

The primary risk factors for cardiovascular disease include:

1) Elevated cholesterol
2) Smoking
3) Diabetes
4) Hypertension
5) Obesity
6) Age
7) Family history
8) Physical inactivity

1. Elevated cholesterol

Cholesterol is a "waxlike substance" that serves as a "building block" within the **cell membrane**.

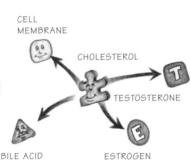

CELL MEMBRANE

CHOLESTEROL

TESTOSTERONE

BILE ACID

ESTROGEN

Cholesterol is used to make **bile acids** that help break down fat in our intestines.

Cholesterol is also used to make **hormones,** especially those found in reproduction: **estrogen** and **testosterone**.

Why is cholesterol so harmful?

As mentioned, **fatty streaks** in the arteries start to develop in the first decade of life as a result of **lipids** moving into the cell wall of the artery. These fatty streaks may become more advanced **atherosclerotic lesions** and may then progress to "advanced lesions" often referred to as **plaque**.

Plaque restricts the flow of blood through the artery, similar to orange construction barrels you have seen on the highway. Plaque reduces the flow of blood (traffic) and increases pressure in the artery (construction zone).

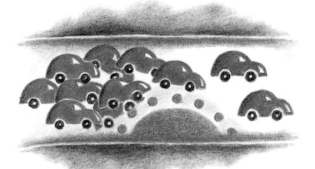

What should my cholesterol levels be?

For those individuals with coronary heart disease or diabetes, **LDL-cholesterol** should be **less than 100 mg/dL**. For individuals with two or more risk factors for cardiovascular disease, **LDL-cholesterol** should be **less than 130 mg/dL**.

Triglycerides should be **less than 200 mg/dL**.

HDL-cholesterol should be **greater than 40 mg/dL** for men and **more than 45 mg/dL** for women.

2. What about smoking?

Don't do it. Smoking is bad for the entire cardiovascular system because it:

A) Introduces carbon monoxide into the body

B) Lowers the "good" HDL-cholesterol

A. Carbon monoxide

Oxygen attaches to the red blood cells in the lungs. Red blood cells transport the oxygen throughout the body.

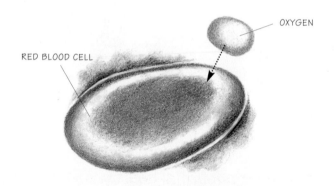

OXYGEN

RED BLOOD CELL

When you smoke, you inhale carbon monoxide into your lungs. Carbon monoxide binds to the red blood cells at the site where oxygen normally binds.

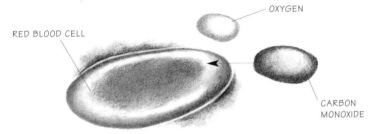

OXYGEN

RED BLOOD CELL

CARBON MONOXIDE

Therefore, less oxygen is carried by the blood, resulting in less oxygen available for use in the heart, muscles, and throughout the body. People who smoke may have abnormal heartbeats as well.

Understandably, smoking has harmful effects, especially for anyone who has already had a heart attack or bypass surgery. More importantly, there is an increased likelihood of a second heart attack or need for another bypass surgery if you continue to smoke after an initial cardiac incident.

Smoking is also a risk factor for peripheral vascular disease (blockages of the arteries to the brain, kidneys and legs).

B. Lower HDL-cholesterol

Two other reasons for not
smoking are that it
reduces the amount of
HDL-cholesterol or
"good cholesterol" in
your bloodstream, and it
makes your blood clot
more easily, increasing
the potential for an
arterial blockage (heart
attack or stroke).

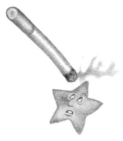

SMOKING
REDUCES
HDL-CHOLESTEROL

39

3. Diabetes

What exactly is diabetes? The working cells need sugar for energy. Sugar is absorbed through the digestive system after a meal or snack. **Insulin** is released by the **pancreas** to allow the body to use sugar as a source of nutrition and energy. That may be hard to visualize. This may help ...

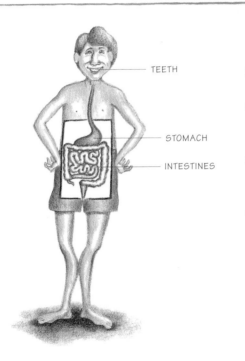

TEETH

STOMACH

INTESTINES

While you eat, the digestive system (teeth, stomach, and intestines) breaks your food down into smaller particles that are used by your body.

41

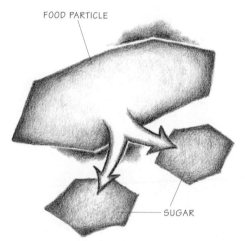

FOOD PARTICLE

SUGAR

Some food is broken down into particles of **sugar**. Sometimes this sugar is referred to as **carbohydrates** or **glucose**.

Sugar moves from the digestive system to the blood and travels throughout the body to feed the working cells. The sugar is the energy packet the cells need to do work like running and breathing.

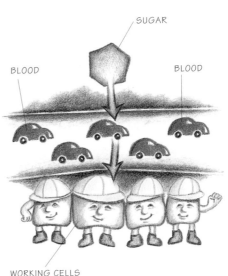

SUGAR

BLOOD

BLOOD

WORKING CELLS

At the same time, the body sends a signal to the **pancreas** telling it to release **insulin** into the bloodstream.

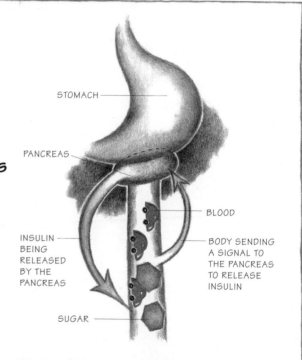

STOMACH

PANCREAS

BLOOD

INSULIN BEING RELEASED BY THE PANCREAS

BODY SENDING A SIGNAL TO THE PANCREAS TO RELEASE INSULIN

SUGAR

Insulin acts like a **key** that unlocks the doors of the cells to let sugar move in. The working cells can then use the sugar for energy to do their jobs. This is how your body uses sugar. However ...

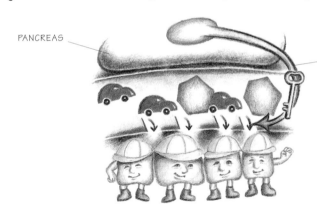

PANCREAS

INSULIN BEING RELEASED BY THE PANCREAS TO ALLOW SUGAR TO MOVE INTO THE WORKING CELLS

Without the key (insulin), the sugar cannot get out of the bloodstream and into the working cells. The sugar builds up in the blood, and the working cells get hungry. This is what happens in diabetes. A diabetic's body cannot move sugar from the blood into the cells.

Diabetes is a major risk factor for cardiovascular disease. Approximately 80% of diabetic patients eventually die of cardiovascular disease. It has been estimated that 50% of diabetics have some form of coronary heart disease prior to being diagnosed with diabetes.

4. Hypertension

SYSTOLIC
NUMBER

140

_____

90

DIASTOLIC
NUMBER

Hypertension is commonly referred to as high blood pressure. If you have a **systolic pressure** greater than 140 mm Hg and/or a **diastolic pressure** greater than 90 mm Hg on 2 separate visits to the doctor, then you may have high blood pressure.

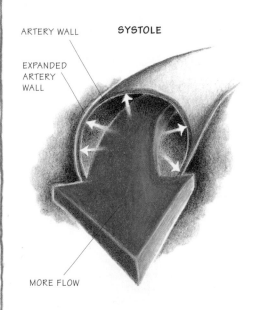

ARTERY WALL

SYSTOLE

EXPANDED
ARTERY
WALL

MORE FLOW

What is **systolic pressure**? Blood comes out of the heart in 1 big thrust. The artery expands to handle the blood. The amount of pressure put on the expanded artery wall is called **systolic pressure**.

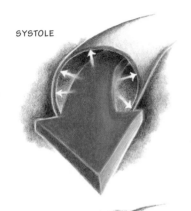

SYSTOLE

After the artery expands during systole, it relaxes back to its normal size. It is similar to a rubber band that goes back to its normal shape after being stretched. Normal pressure on the artery wall during relaxation is called **diastolic pressure**.

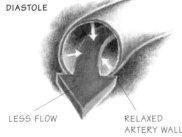

DIASTOLE

LESS FLOW

RELAXED ARTERY WALL

How *does* hypertension relate to cardiovascular disease?

Blood pressure is a result of the blood flowing through the artery (cardiac output) and the resistance of the artery wall (vascular resistance). If that sounds too technical, here ... this may help:

Blood pressure = Cardiac output x vascular resistance

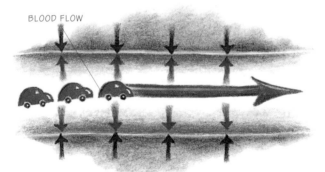

BLOOD FLOW

If a lot of resistance is created by either the blood or the artery wall, then there is more pressure as the blood travels through the artery. If it takes more energy to get the blood through the arteries, then your heart has to work harder with each beat. Most people with high blood pressure do not realize they have it. No wonder hypertension is called the "silent killer."

What contributes to hypertension?

Several factors may contribute to hypertension and cardiovascular disease. These include:

Excess dietary salt
Excess alcohol intake
Stress
Age
Genetics and family history
Obesity
Physical inactivity
High saturated fat diet

Salt

Salt helps conserve water in your body. The American Heart Association Step II Diet recommends that the average person consume no more than 2,400 mg of salt per day, especially those individuals who are salt sensitive. Excess dietary salt may contribute to both hypertension and to your body retaining too much water.

If you are retaining too much water, then you are increasing your blood volume (cars) without adding space. This increase will result in more pressure in the arteries.

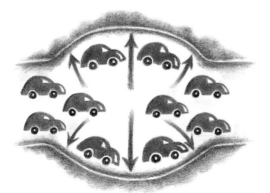

Alcohol consumption

A common concern for individuals with cardiovascular disease is alcohol consumption — mainly because there seems to be conflicting evidence about the benefits versus the risks of drinking. Experts agree that excess alcohol consumption over time can lead to many harmful effects, including high blood pressure, cirrhosis of the liver, and damage to the heart. The issue is the balance between **moderate** and **excessive** alcohol consumption.

While the evidence shows that there is a protective effect for moderate alcohol consumption, this benefit disappears with excessive intake. Men should consume no more than 2 drinks* daily, and women, because of their smaller body size, should not consume more than 1 drink* each day. The 7 to 14 allowable drinks in a week should not be consumed in a few days or during a weekend of binge drinking.

*A guide: One drink is defined as 5 ounces of wine, 12 ounces of beer, or 1-1/2 ounces of 80-proof liquor.

People who should not drink include individuals with high levels of triglycerides in their blood (over 300 mg/dL), women who are pregnant, individuals who are under age, people with a genetic predisposition for alcoholism or who are recovering from alcoholism, and those taking certain medications.

What about stress?

When you are under stress, your brain releases signals to the body through the nerves. These signals allow your body to respond to various situations.

Arteries have nerves attached to them. The nerves can either cause the arteries to relax or can put more tension on the walls of the arteries. If you are under a lot of stress, the nerves send signals to tighten or narrow the arteries.

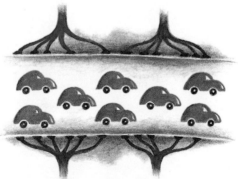

Narrowing the artery is like taking away a lane of traffic. There is still the same number of cars (blood) with less space (artery). This increases the pressure inside the artery.

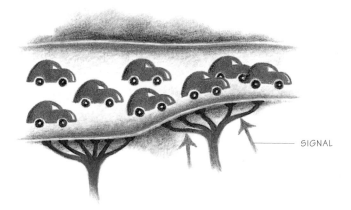

SIGNAL

61

So,

something you can do to improve your blood pressure is reduce stress. You can accomplish this by practicing meditation, doing deep breathing exercises, or doing exercise, such as going for a walk, riding a bike, or taking a swim.

5. Obesity

The American Heart Association has described obesity as a major risk factor for cardiovascular disease. What exactly is obesity?

Metropolitan Life's height/weight tables are often used to determine a recommended weight for an individual based on age and gender. Generally, those who are 20% over the recommended weight for their height are considered to be overweight — but not necessarily obese. Obesity refers to fatness rather than weight. Men who have greater than 25% of their body weight as fat and women who have more than 35% are considered to be obese. Obesity and being overweight carry significant health risks, are directly related to cardiovascular risk factors, and may:

1) raise triglycerides (a "bad" blood fat)
2) lower HDL-cholesterol (the "good" cholesterol)
3) raise LDL-cholesterol (the "bad" cholesterol)
4) raise blood pressure and
5) increase the risk of developing diabetes

Obesity may be related to both genetics (nature) and lifestyle (nurture). Generally speaking, obesity occurs when the calories we consume exceed the calories we burn through activities of daily living and exercise. We store the excess calories as fat reserves, thus contributing to obesity and ultimately increasing the risk of coronary disease. Obesity has increased in men and women in every decade over the past 50 years.

There is a misconception that Americans are overeating and eating too much fat. In fact, as a nation we are eating less fat, fewer calories, and still gaining weight — primarily due to the lower levels of physical activity in our youth and adult lives. A sedentary lifestyle could be the real culprit.

6. Age

Aging has an effect on the risk of cardiovascular disease because aging causes changes in the heart and blood vessels. As people age, they become less active, gain more weight, and the effects of a sedentary lifestyle, smoking, and poor diet continue to damage the heart and circulation by increasing blood pressure and cholesterol levels. Blood pressure increases with aging, in part because arteries gradually lose some of their elasticity and, over time, may not be as resilient.

7. Family history

A **family history** of cardiovascular disease could reflect genetics and/or an unhealthy family lifestyle. If most of your family members smoke, are sedentary, and have a poor diet — then these are harmful habits that increase the risk of heart disease in your family. However, unlike your genes, these behaviors can be changed.

On the other hand, if your family has a healthful lifestyle but there is still a high incidence of cardiovascular disease, then it is likely that genetics is playing a role. We are learning more about the importance of genetic risk for vascular disease. In the future, treatment may be tailored to an individual's own genetic makeup. In either case, by practicing a healthful lifestyle, you can help reduce your risk rather than giving up and thinking you have no control over your destiny.

8. Physical inactivity

Lack of exercise is a major contributor to obesity, diabetes, and hypertension. Beginning an exercise program may help you feel better, help you have more energy, help you lose some weight, lower your cholesterol, lower your blood pressure, help you look better, and improve your muscle tone. Also, beginning an exercise routine can increase your HDL-cholesterol or "good cholesterol" — especially if exercise is associated with weight loss.

Exercise

Currently, only 22% of adults in the United States exercise at a level that benefits their cardiovascular systems. What are some important considerations?

1) Type of exercise

2) Amount and regularity of exercise

3) Intensity of exercise

1. Type of exercise

Aerobic exercise

To meet your general fitness goals, the best type of exercise is **aerobic** exercise.

Aerobic exercise does not necessarily require special equipment or a health club membership. Aerobic exercises are those that require a lot of oxygen. These exercises include walking, jogging, cycling, swimming, cross-country skiing, or rowing.

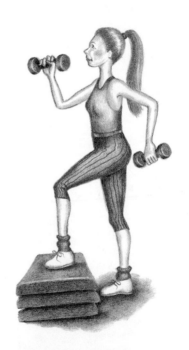

20-30 minutes a day, 5 days a week

2. Amount and regularity of exercise

The U.S. surgeon general recommends that healthy adults exercise 20 to 30 minutes, 5 days a week.

There are nearly 50 half hours in a 24-hour day. Exercising for 30 minutes daily requires **only about 2%** of your total day. Try to find 1, or 2, or 3 exercises you like to do. You'll enjoy the variety.

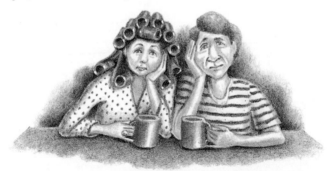

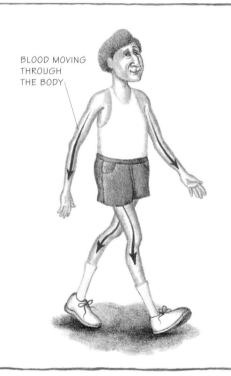

BLOOD MOVING THROUGH THE BODY

3. Intensity of exercise

Warm up

By walking or cycling slowly, you move the blood out to the working muscles. A warm-up should start slowly and last 5 to 10 minutes.

You cannot maintain "all out" exercise (100%) for very long. An example of an "all out" exercise is sprinting. Actually, you may only maintain a sprint for about 15 seconds.

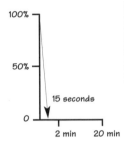

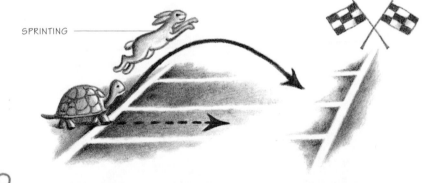

SPRINTING

If you slow the exercise down a bit, to about 90%, you may still only go for about 2 minutes!

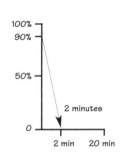

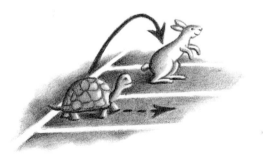

What if you slow your exercise down to 75% or even 50%? There is a **huge** difference. Now you may easily go more than 20 minutes.

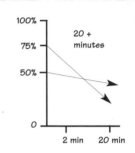

100%

75%

50%

0

20 + minutes

2 min   20 min

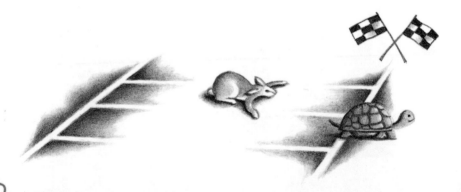

Simply —

By slowing down the pace, you may be able to exercise for a longer period of time.

Many exercise physiologists use the following generally accepted formula to determine the exercise target heart rate of a healthy individual. If you have a history of cardiovascular disease, or if you are just starting a program, **check with your doctor before starting an exercise routine.** Your doctor is aware of the many factors that may need to be considered in modifying your exercise intensity.

Target heart rate example

Your age: 50

Your resting pulse: 70

1. 220 minus your age:
2. Answer #1 minus your resting pulse:
3. Answer #2 times 0.5:
4. Answer #3 plus your resting pulse:
5. Answer #2 times 0.75:
6. Answer #5 plus your resting pulse:
7. **Target heart rate** equals range between values for #4 and #6:

1. $220 - 50 = 170$

2. $170 - 70 = 100$
3. $100 \times 0.5 = 50$

4. $50 + 70 = 120$
5. $100 \times 0.75 = 75$

6. $75 + 70 = 145$
7. **120 to 145 beats per minute, or 12 to 14 beats for 6 seconds**

Now it's your turn

Here is how you determine the heart rate of an apparently healthy individual. Please consult with your doctor to make sure that this is an accurate target heart rate for your condition.

1. Measure your pulse (heart rate) for 60 seconds: _____
2. Take 220 and subtract your age: 220 - _____ = _____
3. Now take the answer in #2 and subtract your pulse: _____
4. Take the answer in #3 and multiply by 0.5: _____
5. Take the answer in #4 and add your pulse: _____
6. Take the answer in #3 and multiply by 0.75: _____
7. Take the answer in #6 and add your pulse: _____
8. Your target heart rate should range from the answer in #5 (_____) to the answer in #7 (_____).
9. Divide each answer in #8 by 10 to determine your pulse for 6 seconds: _____ to _____.

Important!

To begin your exercise program, it may be advantageous for you to exercise only 15 to 20 minutes daily for the first few weeks. This may help you more easily establish a consistent exercise routine. Check with your doctor for input on your exercise program.

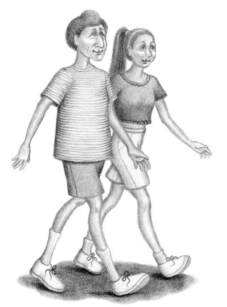

If you are just starting an exercise program, probably the simplest exercise to try is walking. It is fairly easy to do for 20 minutes.

How hard and how often should I exercise?

When you are just starting out, try to exercise very comfortably. Here are 4 quick tips.

1) Try to exercise so that you are breathing noticeably but are **not** out of breath. Remember this simple rule: you should be able to carry on a conversation while you are exercising.

2) Sweating is a good thing. This means that your body is working hard enough and receiving the necessary stimulus for the muscles and the heart.

3) If you are not fatigued and are completely recovered from exercising on the previous day, then you should exercise **daily**.

4) Give yourself a **warm-up** before exercise (several minutes of easy walking) and a **cooldown** at the end of exercise (again, several minutes of easy walking). Ask an exercise specialist for some recommendations for stretching after your workout, and discuss the intensity of the exercise with your doctor.

VERY, VERY important

Cool down. As important as the warm-up and the aerobic exercise are to improving your fitness, you must also include a cooldown as part of your exercise routine.

Your cooldown should be just like your warm-up. At the end of your exercise routine, give yourself 5 to 10 minutes of nice, easy walking. You also may want to include some mild stretching.

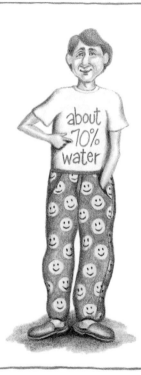

Another consideration — water

Water is needed for virtually every function of the body. The body is approximately 70% water.

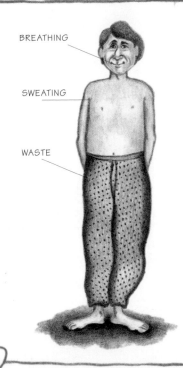

BREATHING

SWEATING

WASTE

During the course of the day, you lose water through sweating, breathing, and waste. Replacement of water (rehydration) is important — especially when participating in an exercise program.

A prudent recommendation is that you should drink 6 to 10 glasses of water per day. Sorry, caffeinated drinks and alcohol do not count. They are "diuretics," meaning that they actually may cause you to lose even more water.

Nutrition

Proper nutrition is an important aspect of our lives — especially for individuals who have heart disease. For example, it is possible to lower your blood cholesterol by changing what you eat. Things that you can do to reduce your cholesterol vary by food group. Start by making changes in one area at a time.

Here's a brief review of the different food groups and a few simple recommendations for healthier eating.

Fats

Not all fats are bad.

Monounsaturated fats are "good" fats. Examples of monounsaturated fats include olive and canola oils, peanut butter, and nuts.

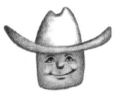

MONOUNSATURATED FAT

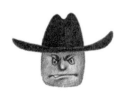

POLYUNSATURATED FAT

Polyunsaturated fats are "acceptable" fats. Examples of polyunsaturated fats include margarine made with corn or safflower oils and some nuts.

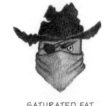

SATURATED FAT

Saturated fats are the "bad" fats, particularly the "**trans**" **fats**. Saturated fats are usually solid at room temperature. Examples of saturated fats include lard, butter, and cream cheese. Examples of "trans" fats include partially hydrogenated vegetable oils found in many snack foods.

It is difficult to eat a diet without saturated fat unless you are on a strict vegetarian diet. While we need fats in our diet, we also need to choose our foods wisely, especially meats, eggs, and dairy products.

People who have had a cardiac event, or people who have high cholesterol and are at risk for cardiovascular disease, should contact a dietitian about reducing their saturated fat intake and limiting their intake of alcohol, caffeine, and salt. The dietitian will also be able to review the amount of sugar you are eating — especially sugars found in "no fat" snack foods.

Meats

As mentioned, limit the amount of fatty meats, particularly those foods that are very high in saturated fats (bacon, sausage, and prime rib), to 1 or 2 servings per week. Cook meats using little or no fat, such as baking, broiling, grilling, stewing, or stir-frying without adding fat. Always trim off the obvious fat **before** cooking red meats and remove the skin before cooking chicken.

TRIM FAT OFF
RED MEAT

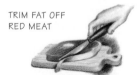

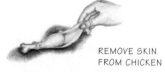

REMOVE SKIN
FROM CHICKEN

Eggs

It used to be thought that these were the main culprits of elevated cholesterol. This may not be true. However, if you have elevated cholesterol or a history of heart disease, you should limit egg yolks to no more than 3 or 4 per week. Egg whites or "egg substitutes" have no cholesterol and do not need to be limited.

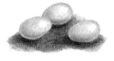

EGGS

Dairy products

Switch from whole milk to 2% and then to 1% or even skim milk. Use low-fat cheeses, yogurt and sour cream. For a healthier dessert, look for low-fat ice cream or sherbet.

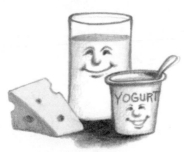

DAIRY PRODUCTS

Whole grains, fruits, and vegetables

Another thing you can do to help improve your overall diet is to eat a variety of healthier foods. The American Heart Association recommends that you try to increase the number of servings of foods that are high in whole grains, such as breads and cereals, and try to have at least **5 servings** of fruits and vegetables every day.

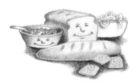

WHOLE GRAINS

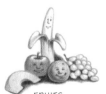

FRUITS

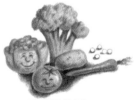

VEGETABLES

What if changing your risk factors, beginning an exercise program, and modifying your diet do not help?

What's next?

Your doctor may refer you to a heart specialist called a **cardiologist**. The cardiologist may have to consider several options including medications or surgical intervention such as **angioplasty** or **bypass surgery**.

Medications, Angioplasty, and Bypass Surgery

Thrombolytics

Most often, a heart attack is caused by a **blood clot** (thrombus) at a site of **atherosclerotic plaque disruption** within the coronary artery. Blood clots can completely block blood flow in the artery and cause a heart attack. If a person gets to a hospital emergency room, usually within 30 minutes of the onset of chest pain, a class of medications called **thrombolytics** may be used to dissolve these clots and restore coronary blood flow. The restoration of blood flow to the heart muscle can save heart muscle and reduce the chance of dying. Thrombolytics are most beneficial if given soon after the onset of heart attack symptoms.

Certain individuals may not be candidates to receive thrombolytics, including individuals who have had a recent stroke, surgery, or trauma that would increase the risk of serious bleeding. Likewise, individuals with bleeding peptic ulcers, very high blood pressure, or very advanced age may be at increased risk with thrombolytic therapy. An alternative treatment to thrombolytic therapy for a heart attack is **coronary angioplasty**.

Angioplasty

Angioplasty is a procedure by which the cardiologist inserts a balloon catheter over a thin wire across a blockage of a coronary artery.

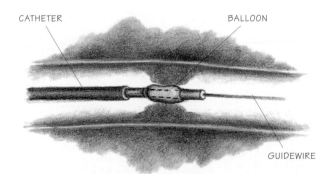

CATHETER

BALLOON

GUIDEWIRE

The balloon is inflated to compress the plaque.
This is repeated as necessary by the cardiologist.

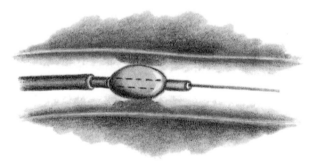

Inflating the catheter compresses and breaks apart the plaque. This allows more room for the blood to flow.

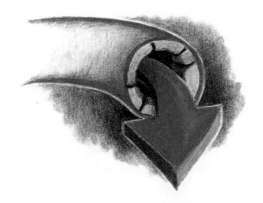

The balloon catheter also stretches the elastic wall of the artery. Small tears occur on the inside of the artery wall and slightly injure the artery wall as a result of balloon catheter inflation.

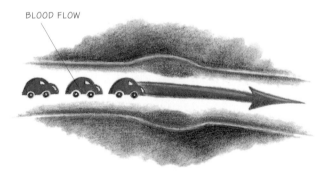

BLOOD FLOW

Unfortunately, these balloon catheter injuries expose substances from inside the atherosclerotic plaque and the artery wall that promote formation of blood clots. Complications of this procedure may include a heart attack, repeat angioplasty, the need for emergency coronary bypass surgery, and even death.

Stents

In certain instances, the cardiologist may decide to insert a **stent** inside the coronary artery. The stent, usually made of stainless steel, functions as a scaffold to hold open the inside of the coronary artery.

STENT

Stents are usually put in place using a balloon angioplasty catheter. Stents can reduce the incidence of both 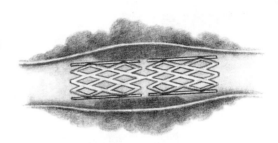 short- and long-term coronary artery reocclusion. Stents can seal and "tack up" tissue flaps within the artery that are created when a balloon catheter injures the artery. Unfortunately, stents do not eliminate clot formation or the occurrence of heart attack following the procedure.

What can be done to reduce blood clot formation and reduce the risk of reocclusion?

Antiplatelet therapy

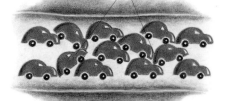

BLOOD PLATELETS "STICKING TOGETHER"

After angioplasty, the blood platelets may be susceptible to "sticking together" and forming clots. To reduce this likelihood, cardiologists have historically administered aspirin and a drug called heparin before and after angioplasty. Although these medicines have been shown to reduce the chance of clot formation during and after angioplasty, they have limited effectiveness. Newer medications have been developed to further improve results.

Improved outcomes

A class of medicines called IIb/IIIa receptor blockers has been developed that reduces blood clot formation during

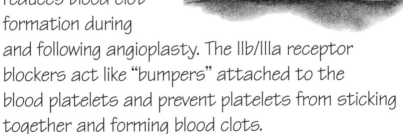

"BUMPERS" ATTACHED TO THE BLOOD PLATELETS

and following angioplasty. The IIb/IIIa receptor blockers act like "bumpers" attached to the blood platelets and prevent platelets from sticking together and forming blood clots.

Bypass surgery

Bypass surgery is a cardiovascular procedure designed to correct blood flow to the heart that angioplasty cannot correct. The cardiovascular surgeon uses a piece of artery and/or vein to reroute blood around the blockage.

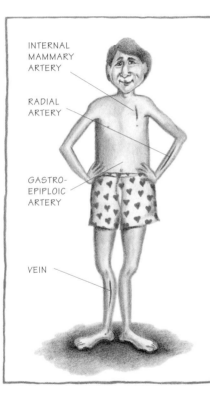

INTERNAL MAMMARY ARTERY

RADIAL ARTERY

GASTRO-EPIPLOIC ARTERY

VEIN

The surgeon may use a vein from the leg, and/or the internal mammary artery found in the chest, and/or the gastroepiploic artery of the stomach, and/or the radial artery of the forearm.

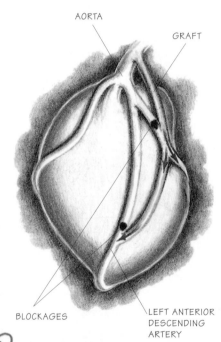

AORTA

GRAFT

BLOCKAGES

LEFT ANTERIOR
DESCENDING
ARTERY

The vein is attached
to the aorta. The supply
of blood is then rerouted
around the blockage. One
piece of vein may be used
for multiple bypasses.
The number of blockages
where blood has been
rerouted — not the
number of veins used —
determines the number
of bypasses.

If the internal mammary artery is used, the artery originates from a branch off the aorta and is attached directly below the blockage.

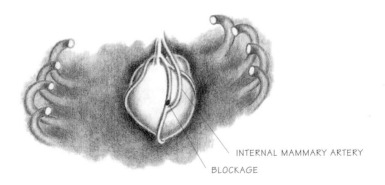

INTERNAL MAMMARY ARTERY

BLOCKAGE

What about 'after care' from a heart attack, bypass surgery, or angioplasty?

Your doctor will manage your care very closely. Generally, the cardiologist may recommend that you:

- quit smoking
- take a beta blocker drug (after a heart attack)
- lower your LDL-cholesterol below 100 mg/dL
- take a daily enteric-coated aspirin (81 mg or greater) unless you have other medical complications
- follow a "heart-healthy diet" and begin a basic exercise program, mainly walking. Always follow your doctor's recommendations.

Questions

Here are some questions that you may want to take with you the next time you go to see your doctor.

What are my medications? How does each of them help me?

Answer _____

_____

_____

_____

_____

_____

_____

123

List the blood pressure reading for each visit to your doctor and the date:

Date	Blood Pressure
_____	_____
_____	_____
_____	_____
_____	_____
_____	_____
_____	_____

List the total cholesterol (TC), LDL-cholesterol (LDL), triglycerides (Trig), and HDL-cholesterol (HDL) readings for each visit to your doctor.

Date	TC	LDL	Trig	HDL
____	____	____	____	____
____	____	____	____	____
____	____	____	____	____
____	____	____	____	____
____	____	____	____	____
____	____	____	____	____

Do I have any exercise limitations of which I should be aware? What are they?

Answer _____

_____

Should I have a treadmill test before I start to exercise? What is my target heart rate?

Answer _____

_____

Based on my weight, blood pressure, and blood cholesterol level, should I talk to someone about changing my diet?

Yes   No

Contact your local hospital for the name of a registered dietitian.

Dietitian _____

Address _____

_____

Phone _____

Are there any concerns that I should be aware of before having/resuming sexual activity?

Answer

_____

_____

_____

_____

And now for a little
heart to heart ...

It has been mentioned throughout the book, but the importance of seeing your doctor and having a complete physical exam cannot be stressed enough. If necessary, sit down with a dietitian and review your current eating pattern. Then, if your doctor agrees, get moving. Start a simple exercise program — mainly walking. There are no guarantees you will reduce your risk of having a cardiac event, but at least you will be taking an aggressive approach to improving your health.

Bibliography

American College of Sports Medicine position stand. "The Recommended Quality and
    Quantity of Exercise for Developing and Maintaining Cardiorespiratory and Muscular
    Fitness in Healthy Adults." *Medicine and Science in Sports and Exercise* April 1990.

Angell, M. "Caring for women's health – What is the problem?" *New England Journal of
    Medicine* 1993: 271.

Burke, A.P., and A. Farb, G.T. Malcom, Y. Liang, J. Smialek, R. Virmani. "Coronary Risk
    Factors and Plaque Morphology in Men with Coronary Disease Who Died Suddenly."
    New England Journal of Medicine 1 May 1997: 1276-1282.

Cogswell, M.E. "Nicotine Withdrawal Symptoms." *North Carolina Medical Journal* 1 Jan. 1995: 40-45.

Collins, R., and R. Peto, C. Baigent, P. Sleight. "Aspirin, Heparin, and Fibrinolytic Therapy in Suspected
    Acute Myocardial Infarction." *New England Journal of Medicine* 20 March 1997: 847-860.

Da Costa, F.D., et al. "Myocardial Revascularization with the Radial Artery: A Clinical and
    Angiographic Study." *Annals of Thoracic Surgery* Aug. 1996: 475-480.

Eckel, R.H. "Obesity in Heart Disease." *Circulation* 1997: 3248-3250.

Executive Summary of the Third Report of the National Cholesterol Education Program (NCEP)
    Expert Panel on Detection, Evaluation, and Treatment of High Blood Cholesterol in Adults
    (Adult Treatment Panel III). JAMA, May 16, 2001, Vol. 285, No. 19: 2486-2497.

Friedman, G.D., and A.L. Klatsky. "Is Alcohol Good for Your Health?" *New England Journal
    of Medicine* 16 Dec. 1993: 1882-1883.

131

Gellar, A. "Common Addictions." *Clinical Symposia*. Ciba-Geigy Corporation 1996.

Grossman, E., and F.H. Messerli. "Diabetic and Hypertensive Heart Disease." *Annals of Internal Medicine* 15 Aug. 1996: 304-310.

Henningfield, J.D., and R.M. Keenan. "The Anatomy of Nicotine Addiction." *Health Values* March/April 1993: 12-19.

Joint National Committee. The Fifth Report of the Joint National Committee on Detection, Evaluation, and Treatment of High Blood Pressure. Bethesda (MD): National Institutes of Health, National Heart, Lung, and Blood Institute; 1993. NIH publication No. 93-1008.

Kannel, W.B., and R.B. D'Agostino, J.L. Cobb. "Effects of Weight on Cardiovascular Disease." *American Journal of Clinical Nutrition* March 1996: 419S-422S.

Kenney, W.L. et al. *American College of Sports Medicine Guidelines for Exercise Testing and Prescription*. 5th ed. Media, Pa.: Williams & Wilkins, 1995.

Margolis, S., and P.J. Goldschmidt-Clermont. *The Johns-Hopkins White Papers*. Baltimore: The Johns-Hopkins Medical Institutions, 1996.

McCarron, D.A., and M.E. Reusser. "Body Weight and Blood Pressure Regulation." *American Journal of Clinical Nutrition* March 1996: 423S-425S.

Meeker, M.H., and J.C. Rothrock. *Alexander's Care of the Patient in Surgery*, 10th ed. St. Louis: Mosby, 1995.

Peterson, J.A., and C.X. Bryant, *The Fitness Handbook; 2nd edition*, St. Louis: Wellness Bookshelf, 1995.

Ryan, T.J., and J.L. Anderson, E.M. Autman, et al. "ACC/AHA Guidelines for the Management of Patients with Acute Myocardial Infarction: A Report of the American College of Cardiology/American Heart Association Task Force on Practice Guidelines (Committee on Management of Acute Myocardial Infarction)." *Journal of the American College of Cardiology* 1 Nov. 1996: 1328-1428.

St. Jeor, S.T., and K.D. Brownell, R.L. Atkinson, C. Bouchard, et al. "Obesity Workshop III." *Circulation* 1996: 1391-1396.

Schlant, R.C., and R.W. Alexander. *The Heart*, 8th ed. New York: McGraw-Hill, 1994.

Superko, H.R. "The Most Common Cause of Coronary Heart Disease can be Successfully Treated by the Least Expensive Therapy — Exercise." *Certified News* 1998: 1-5.

United States Surgeon General. Department of Health and Human Services. *The Health Consequences of Smoking. Nicotine Addiction.* Washington, D.C.: U.S. Department of Health and Human Services, 1988.

United States Surgeon General on his priorities at http://www.osophs.dhhs.gov/myjob/priorities.htm accessed November 1999.

Voors, A.A., et al. "Smoking and Cardiac Events After Venous Coronary Bypass Surgery." *Circulation* Jan 1, 1995: 42-47.

Voutilainen, S., et al. "Angiographic 5-Year Follow-up Study of Right Gastroepiploic Artery Grafts." *Annals of Thoracic Surgery* Aug. 1996: 501-505.

White H.D., and J.J. Van de Werf. "Thrombolysis for Acute Myocardial Infarction." *Circulation* 28 April 1998: 1632-1646.

Zelasko, C.J. "Exercise for Weight Loss: What are the Facts?" *Journal of the American Dietetic Association* Dec. 1995: 973-1031.

Notes

Notes

About the Authors

Dean J. Kereiakes, MD, FACC, is one of the nation's preeminent cardiologists. Dr. Kereiakes is President of the Ohio Heart Health Center; Medical Director of the Carl and Edyth Linder Center for Clinical Cardiovascular Research; Professor of Clinical Medicine at the University of Cincinnati; and Professor of Medicine at The Ohio State University. He frequently lectures worldwide and has published hundreds of articles and papers. Dr. Kereiakes lives in Cincinnati, Ohio.

Douglas Wetherill, MS, is Supervisor of Disease Management at a large Midwest manufacturing company. He lives in Cincinnati, Ohio.

For additional copies of *Heart Disease: What You Should Know*™, please contact your local bookseller or call (800) 216-2522

For institutional quantities, contact our Special Sales Department at rsimet@blacksci.com or call (800) 759-6102

Other titles in the series *Your Health: What You Should Know*™:

Congestive Heart Failure: What You Should Know™
Diabetes: What You Should Know™
High Cholesterol: What You Should Know™
Women's Health Over 40: What You Should Know™
Women's Health Under 40: What You Should Know™